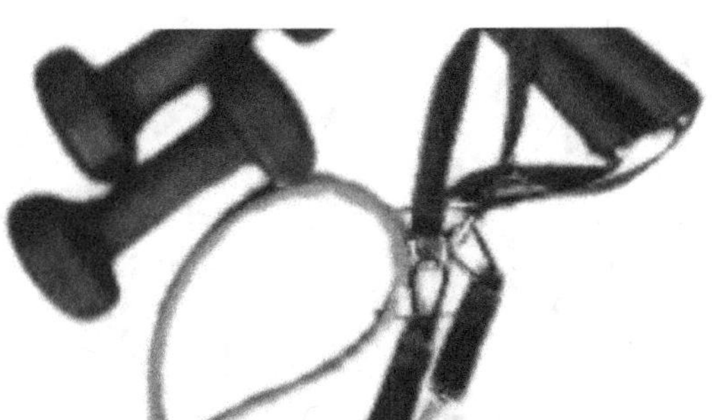

KEGEL EXERCISES
for
ERECTILE DYSFUNCTION

Your Complete Step-by-step Guide to Ending ED, Get Your Erections Back, Overcome Impotence, and Improve Sexual Health

THERESA BELLS

KEGEL EXERCISES FOR ERECTILE DYSFUNCTION

Your Complete Step-by-step Guide to Ending ED, Get Your Erections Back, Overcome Impotence, and Improve Sexual Health

Theresa Bells

<u>DISCLAIMER</u>

The information provided in 'Kegel Exercises for Erectile Dysfunction' is for educational purposes only and should not replace professional medical advice. Readers are advised to consult with healthcare professionals before starting any new exercise regimen, especially if dealing with underlying health conditions. The author and publisher are not liable for any consequences arising from the use of the information in this book.

Table of Contents

"Strength isn't just measured in the muscles we see; it's also in the ones we nurture silently. Kegel exercises—the quiet strength of a vibrant connection."

Introduction

Meet Larry. Larry sat in his dimly lit living room, feeling pretty resigned as the evening light faded away. His marriage, which used to be full of passion and connection, was now struggling because of a silent problem – erectile dysfunction. The spark in their relationship had faded, and Larry was dealing with not just a physical issue but also a big emotional gap that seemed impossible to fix.

During one of his lowest moments, when he was feeling super frustrated and down, Larry found a solution that changed his life: Kegel exercises. At first, he wasn't sure about it, but he did some research and found out that these exercises were not just for women; they could help men too. Larry was determined to get back what he had lost, so he started a routine of pelvic health exercises.

As Larry kept doing Kegels, something amazing happened. Each exercise made a small but really important change in him. His pelvic floor muscles got stronger, and, more importantly, he began to feel more confident and in control. It wasn't just about fixing erectile dysfunction; it was about getting back his energy, his connection with his own body, and, most importantly, fixing his marriage.

Larry worked hard and saw a big change. His marriage, which was almost falling apart, got better. The intimacy he thought was gone came back, not just physically but emotionally and spiritually too. Kegel exercises became more than just a routine for Larry; they became the thing that helped him start over, giving him a new chance at a better life than he ever thought possible.

Kegel exercises have been a game-changer for thousands of people, and Larry's story is just one of many. Lots of marriages and relationships have been saved by this simple but revolutionary exercise.

You can learn everything about it in this book. "Kegel Exercises for Erectile Dysfunction" isn't just a guide; it's a story about how each of us can make a big change in our lives, get our energy back, and bring back the passion and connection in our relationships.

"Reclaiming confidence isn't just about lifting weights; sometimes, it's about the strength you build from within with Kegel exercises."

Chapter 1: Understanding Erectile Dysfunction

Erectile Dysfunction (ED) can be a problem for many men, making it hard for them to have and keep an erection. It's important to know why this happens to treat it well. Sometimes, it's normal to have trouble getting or keeping an erection, but if it happens a lot, there might be a bigger issue.

ED has different causes, and they often connect. One main cause is not enough blood going to the penis. Conditions like atherosclerosis, which makes arteries narrow and hard, can stop the right blood flow for a good erection. High blood pressure and diabetes, which are common problems, can also hurt blood vessels and nerves, making the issue worse.

Hormone problems also matter. Testosterone, a hormone important for male sex, can be messed up by diseases like hypogonadism. To fix ED, it's important to deal with hormone issues.

Things in the mind are a big part too. Stress, worry, and feeling sad can mess up the brain signals needed for an erection. Being nervous about performance is common and can make ED happen more.

What you do in your life matters too. Smoking, drinking too much alcohol, and using drugs can hurt blood vessels and nerves, affecting how well you can get hard. Not being active and being too heavy both make your heart health bad, which is a big reason for ED.

Also, some medicines can make ED happen. Pills for feeling sad, high blood pressure, and prostate problems are usual ones. Talking to a healthcare person about different medicine options is important.

Understanding all the things that cause ED helps you make smart choices for your health. Getting help from a professional is a good move to take control of your sexual health. A healthcare person can look at everything to figure out what's causing your ED and make a plan just for you.

Doing things to fix the causes of ED is a good way to get healthier overall. Eating foods that are good for your heart, doing regular exercise, and handling stress are changes you can make. Also, getting help for any problems in your mind is part of taking care of ED in a complete way.

In the end, knowing why ED happens is a big first step. It means understanding how your body, mind, and what you do all work together. By facing these things, you can control your sexual health and find good answers.

Impact on Quality of Life

Erectile Dysfunction (ED) goes beyond being just a medical issue; it affects more than just how someone feels emotionally or their general well-being. The emotional impact of ED on people and their relationships can be big and varied.

The struggle with self-esteem is a big part of how ED emotionally affects someone. Men dealing with ED often battle with feelings of not being good enough and dissatisfaction. Society saying that being virile means being manly only makes these feelings worse. It's important to know that having ED doesn't make someone less valuable or masculine, but societal ideas can make someone feel bad about themselves.

The emotional burden isn't only on the person dealing with ED; it also affects their relationships. Partners might feel rejected or blame themselves for their loved one's condition. Open and understanding communication is the key to dealing with these emotional challenges. Partners should be encouraged to talk about their thoughts and feelings, creating a supportive atmosphere.

Many relationships depend on intimacy, and ED can affect that part of a relationship. Worrying about not performing well can lead to avoiding intimacy and making the problem worse. Breaking this cycle requires open communication, patience, and both partners committing to finding solutions. Getting professional help, either alone or as a couple, can provide helpful advice and strategies for dealing with these emotional hurdles.

Aside from the emotional stress, ED might be a sign of bigger health problems. The same issues causing ED could also mean there are problems with the heart. Looking at ED as a sign of overall health, not just a sexual issue, is a broader way of thinking about well-being.

Changing ideas about what it means to be masculine and building individual and relationship strength are two ways to handle the emotional impact of ED. People should learn to see their value beyond sexual performance, recognizing all the qualities that make them special.

Partners also play a big role in creating a positive environment. Understanding that ED is something both partners deal with, not just one person's problem, builds understanding and strengthens the emotional connection. Trying different ways of being intimate can also help reduce the stress of sexual performance.

Getting professional help is a good step in lessening the emotional impact of ED. Mental health professionals and sex therapists can guide individuals and couples through the emotional challenges of ED, offering ways to cope and communicate better. Including therapy in the overall plan recognizes how physical and emotional well-being are connected.

Understanding How Kegel Exercises Contribute to Treatment for Erectile Dysfunction

Let's take a closer look at a potential method for addressing erectile dysfunction (ED): the incorporation of Kegel exercises. While these exercises are commonly associated with women's health, they have garnered attention for their potential benefits in assisting men with ED. To grasp their role in ED treatment, it's essential to look into the anatomy involved.

The pelvic floor muscles, often overlooked, play a pivotal role in sexual function for both men and women. These muscles provide essential support to pelvic organs, including the bladder, rectum, and notably, the prostate. By strengthening these muscles, it is believed that blood flow to the genital area can be improved, potentially enhancing erectile function.

For men, these pelvic floor muscles are crucial in various aspects of sexual health. They contribute to the achievement and maintenance of erections, control ejaculation, and support overall sexual satisfaction. Weakness in these muscles may contribute to ED, leading us to the relevance of Kegel exercises.

Kegels primarily target the pubococcygeus (PC) muscle, a hammock-like muscle extending from the pubic bone to the coccyx. Locating this muscle is the initial step in performing Kegel exercises. An easy way to identify it is by interrupting the flow of urine midstream, engaging the PC muscle. However, it's crucial to note that Kegels should not be practiced during regular urination, as this may result in incomplete bladder emptying.

Once the PC muscle is identified, Kegel exercises can be introduced into a daily routine. The fundamental technique involves contracting the PC muscle for a few seconds and then releasing it. Gradually increasing the duration and repetitions over time aims to enhance muscle strength, and consistency is key to experiencing the full benefits.

The potential advantages of Kegel exercises for ED are rooted in their ability to promote blood circulation, strengthen pelvic floor muscles, and enhance overall sexual function. Research suggests that incorporating Kegels into a comprehensive ED treatment plan may yield positive outcomes, particularly when combined with other lifestyle modifications.

However, it's crucial to approach Kegel exercises as part of a broader strategy. Maintaining a healthy weight, engaging in regular exercise, and adopting a balanced diet significantly contribute to erectile health. Furthermore, addressing the underlying causes of ED, such as cardiovascular problems or hormonal imbalances, is critical for comprehensive, long-term management.

Before embarking on a Kegel exercise routine, seeking guidance from a healthcare professional is advisable. They can offer personalized advice, ensuring that Kegels are a suitable addition to an individual's treatment plan. Additionally, proper technique is vital to minimize potential issues, such as overworking the muscles.

The role of Kegel exercises in ED treatment holds promise, providing a non-invasive and accessible option for improving pelvic floor muscle strength. As with any aspect of health, individual responses may vary, and it's important to approach Kegels as part of a comprehensive strategy.

Chapter 2: Anatomy and Physiology

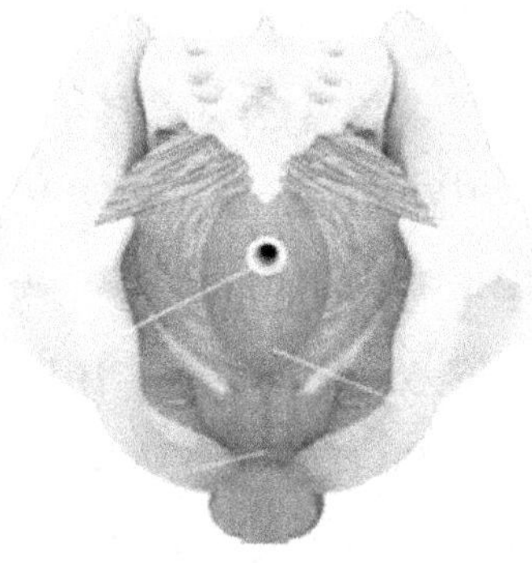

The male reproductive system is a network of parts that work together for making and moving sperm. It's not just for making babies, but it also affects overall health.

Testes: The testes are two small glands in the scrotum that make sperm. They need to be a bit cooler than the body, so the scrotum keeps them that way. Inside the testes, tiny tubes work hard to produce sperm in a process called spermatogenesis.

Epididymis: New sperm go through the epididymis, a coiled tube on each testis. During sex, sperm mature here and get ready to fertilize an egg. The epididymis is like a waiting room for sperm before they move to the next stop.

Vas Deferens: The vas deferens is a tube that connects the epididymis to the urethra. Its job during ejaculation is to carry mature sperm to the urethra. Before reaching the urethra, it mixes with fluids from the seminal vesicles and prostate gland that help the sperm. **Seminal Vesicles and Prostate Gland:** These guys provide fluids that support sperm survival and movement. Seminal vesicles give most of the liquid in semen, along with energy for the sperm. The prostate gland adds a milky fluid that helps the sperm survive.

Urethra: The urethra runs from the bladder to the penis, doing two jobs for the reproductive and urine systems. It carries sperm out during ejaculation and lets urine out from the bladder.

Penis: The penis has two jobs: pleasure and reproduction. Blood flow increases during arousal, leading to an erection. This helps with penetration during sex, letting sperm enter the female reproductive canal.

Erectile Dysfunction and Kegel Exercises

Understanding how the male reproductive system works is crucial for dealing with issues like erectile dysfunction (ED). ED happens when a man can't get or keep a good erection for sex, and it can be caused by things like age, health conditions, or mental issues.

Kegel exercises, often linked to women's health, are now seen as helpful for men with ED. These exercises focus on the pelvic floor muscles, important for sexual function. The main muscle worked is called the pubococcygeus (PC) muscle.

Men can make the PC muscle stronger, boost blood flow to the pelvic area, and improve erections by doing Kegel exercises regularly. These exercises also help with controlling ejaculation and can benefit those with premature ejaculation.

Every part of the male reproductive system plays a unique role in making reproduction and sex work well. Knowing how these parts function helps us explore treatments like Kegel exercises for conditions like erectile dysfunction. As we dig into the world of male sexual health, we see how targeted exercises can be a complete approach to overcoming challenges and improving overall well-being.

Chapter 3: Getting to Know Kegel Exercises

Kegel exercises are a straightforward but effective method for boosting erectile function. In this chapter, we'll cover the basics, looking at what Kegel exercises is, their origin, and how they might be your secret weapon in tackling erectile dysfunction.

Understanding Kegel Exercises

Let's demystify Kegel exercises. These exercises, named after Dr. Arnold Kegel, introduced in the 1940s, aim to strengthen the pelvic floor muscles. But where exactly is this pelvic floor? Think of it as the center of your body, supporting vital organs and playing a crucial role in controlling the bladder and bowel.

The pelvic floor muscles are like the unsung heroes of your body, often unnoticed until issues arise. They form a hammock-like structure between your tailbone and pubic bone. Picture these muscles as a rubber band: flexible yet sturdy.

Kegel exercises focus on the pubococcygeus (PC) muscles, part of the pelvic floor group. These muscles control urine flow, aid in bowel movements, and, importantly for humans, contribute to sexual function. When weakened, they can lead to various issues, including erectile dysfunction.

So, how do you perform Kegel exercises? The beauty lies in their simplicity. Pause the flow of urine midstream to locate the PC muscles – these are the muscles you'll be working on. Remember, though, don't do Kegels while urinating regularly, as it may result in incomplete bladder emptying.

Once you've pinpointed your PC muscles, start integrating Kegel exercises into your routine. Begin by contracting these muscles for three counts, then relaxing for three counts. Repeat this cycle 10 times, gradually increasing the duration as your muscles get stronger.

Benefits of Kegel Exercises for Men

Starting Kegel exercises is more than just a commitment; it's an investment in your overall well-being, especially when dealing with erectile dysfunction. Let's explore the fantastic list of advantages that you can enjoy:

1. Relief from Erectile Dysfunction: Kegel exercises boost blood flow to the pelvic area, improving erectile function. Strengthening the pelvic floor muscles provides better support for the blood vessels and nerves related to sexual function.

2. Better Sexual Performance: Think of your pelvic floor muscles as key players in the stage of intimacy. Strengthening them through Kegel exercises enhances your strength, control, and endurance, allowing you to lead in the performance and ensuring a memorable experience for both you and your partner.

3. Increased Orgasmic Sensation: Learning Kegel exercises gives you more control over your pelvic floor muscles, intensifying orgasms. This newfound control enhances pleasure and extends bliss, turning your private moments into a more enjoyable experience.

4. Bladder Control: Beyond sexual health, Kegel exercises offer another important benefit: improved bladder control. Strengthening pelvic floor muscles can help with issues like incontinence, letting you engage in activities without worrying about leaks.

5. Prostate Health: Kegel exercises are good for prostate health. They promote a healthy prostate by increasing blood flow and strengthening muscles in the pelvic area, reducing the risk of prostate-related problems.

6. Prevention of Premature Ejaculation: Kegel exercises help you manage the timing of pelvic contractions, naturally combating premature ejaculation. With practice, you can learn to delay ejaculation, leading to a more satisfying and prolonged experience for both you and your partner.

7. Increased Confidence: Learning Kegel exercises has a crucial but often overlooked effect—an increase in confidence. Actively contributing to your sexual health can boost confidence in both intimate and daily situations.

Now that you know about the many benefits awaiting you, let's focus on the practical aspects of incorporating Kegel exercises into your daily routine.

Starting with Kegels

Kegel exercises are a fantastic way to boost your health and well-being. Let's get started with incorporating these exercises into your daily routine.

1. Find Your Muscles: Take a moment to locate your pelvic floor muscles before diving into a full Kegel program. Just like stopping the flow of pee midstream, these are the muscles you use. Once you've found them, practice contracting and releasing until you get the hang of it.

2. Set a Schedule: Consistency is key in any exercise plan. Pick a specific time each day for your Kegel exercises—whether it's in the morning, during your commute, or before bedtime. Regularity ensures you get the full benefits of this exercise.

3. Begin Gradually: If you're new to Kegel exercises, start with short contractions and relaxations. Aim for three-second contractions and three-second relaxations. Increase the duration as your muscles gain strength.

4. Repeat Regularly: Like lifting weights, building strength with Kegels requires repetition. Aim for three sets of ten repetitions each day. Focus on quality over quantity, making each contraction deliberate and controlled.

5. Add Variety: Keep things interesting by trying different types of Kegel exercises. Experiment with fast contractions followed by slow releases or holding contractions for a longer time. This variety targets different aspects of your pelvic floor muscles.

6. Integrate into Daily Activities: One of the perks of Kegel exercises is their flexibility.

Easily include them in your daily routines—
whether sitting at your desk, watching TV, or
waiting in line. It'll become second nature over
time.

7. Be Patient and Positive: Results may
take time, so stay patient. Celebrate small
successes along the way, recognizing your
efforts and positive changes. Positive
reinforcement is a great motivator.

8. Get Professional Guidance: If you're
unsure about doing Kegel exercises correctly or
have specific health concerns, consult a
healthcare practitioner or physical therapist.
They can offer personalized advice to ensure
you're on the right track.

Incorporating Kegel exercises into your routine
is a long-term commitment to your health.
Remember, you're investing in a healthier,
more confident version of yourself, beyond just
your pelvic floor muscles.

Facing Common Challenges in Kegel Exercises

Starting Kegel exercises is a good choice, but it has its challenges, like any important goal. Let's look at common issues and tips to overcome them for a smooth and successful experience with Kegels.

Inconsistency: Life can be busy, and adding another workout routine may seem hard. The key is to include Kegel exercises in your regular schedule. Do them regularly, whether with your morning coffee, on your way to work, or before bedtime. Consistency is crucial, and it doesn't have to be complicated.

Lack of Motivation: Staying motivated when you don't see instant results can be tough. Set realistic goals and celebrate small achievements. Keep track of your progress, noting improvements in endurance or the ability to hold contractions longer. Sharing your goals with a friend or partner can provide the support you need.

Difficulty Identifying Muscles: Some people may struggle to isolate and contract their pelvic floor muscles. If you're having trouble, consider consulting a doctor or a physical therapist for guidance. They can ensure you're targeting the right muscles and tailor your program to address any specific issues.

Excessive Exertion: While enthusiasm is great, overworking your pelvic floor muscles can cause fatigue or pain. Start with shorter contractions and gradually increase length and intensity. Pushing your muscles too hard may not be as beneficial as doing controlled contractions.

Mind-Body Connection: Developing the mind-body connection for effective Kegel exercises takes time. Be patient and practice mindfulness. Pay attention to the sensations in your pelvic area during contractions and relaxations. Visualization techniques, like imagining your pelvic floor muscles as a strong hammock, can help strengthen this connection.

Distractions: Distractions are common in our fast-paced lives. Finding a quiet, comfortable place to practice and turning off notifications can help maintain focus. Use this time for mindfulness and relaxation.

Incorporating Variety: Doing the same routine every day can lead to boredom. As mentioned before, try different variations to keep it interesting. Experiment with varied contraction and relaxation periods, and explore how different postures affect pelvic floor muscle involvement.

Patience in Results: The benefits of Kegel exercises may take time to show. Be patient and focus on the journey rather than the destination. Celebrate your achievements along the way. Building pelvic floor strength requires time and consistency.

By overcoming these challenges, you not only enhance your physical strength but also build mental resilience. Embrace the journey, adapt to setbacks, and stay committed to positive changes in your life. Your dedication to overcoming obstacles in Kegel exercises reflects your commitment to a healthier, more vibrant self. Keep going—the rewards are worth it!

Chapter 4: Discovering Pelvic Floor Muscles

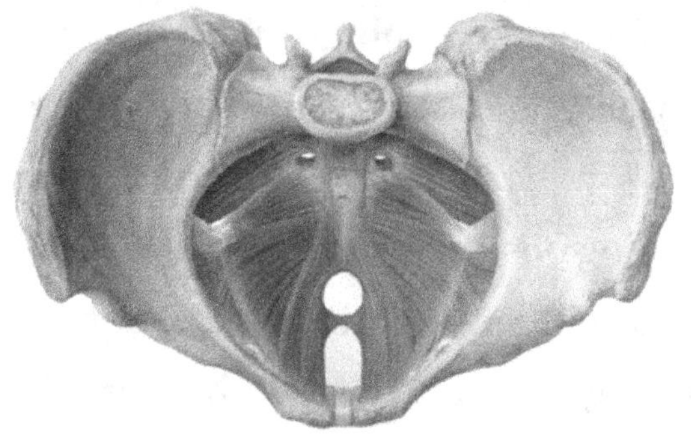

Knowing about the muscles that help your pelvic organs, like the bladder and uterus, is the first thing to do in understanding your pelvic floor muscles. These muscles, which people sometimes don't think about, do an important job in controlling pee and poop, and also help support important organs.

Learning about and getting to know these muscles is really important for keeping your pelvic area healthy and preventing issues like peeing when you don't want to or organs moving out of place.

Locating the Pelvic Floor Muscles

Initiating the quest to overcome erectile dysfunction with Kegel exercises requires a heightened awareness of your pelvic floor muscles. Despite their discreet presence, these muscles play a pivotal role in sexual function and can be intentionally managed and strengthened through focused workouts.

What and Where are the Pelvic Floor Muscles?

Situated at the base of your pelvis, your pelvic floor muscles form a sling-like structure, providing support to your pelvic organs and aiding in bladder and bowel control. To identify these elusive muscles, visualize the act of halting the flow of urine midstream. Your pelvic floor muscles come into play during this deliberate action.

Feeling the Pelvic Floor

A Hands-On Approach Employing touch is an additional effective method for locating these muscles. Find a serene and comfortable environment. Relax your muscles, focus on your breath while lying down or sitting, and gently insert a clean, lubricated finger into your rectum. Simulate the act of squeezing or lifting your finger. The muscles contracting around your finger are your pelvic floor muscles.

Understanding Muscle Engagement

It is crucial to comprehend the subtleties of engaging your pelvic floor muscles as you identify them. Instead of pushing or bearing down, the contraction should entail a gentle lift and squeeze. Envision pushing these muscles upward and inward, as if you are endeavoring to move them away from the surface you are seated on. This upward motion is fundamental for the success of Kegel exercises.

Practical Tips for Locating Muscles

Diversify your muscle identification exercises by practicing in various positions—lying down, sitting, and standing. Commence with brief contractions to prevent muscular fatigue. During the identification process, refrain from activating adjacent muscles such as the abdominal or buttock muscles.

The Significance of Muscle Awareness

The cornerstone for effective Kegel exercises lies in developing a heightened awareness of your pelvic floor muscles. This increased awareness not only amplifies the efficacy of the workouts but also empowers you to confidently address and overcome concerns related to erectile dysfunction.

You have taken a significant stride towards reclaiming control of your sexual health by acquiring the technique to locate your pelvic floor muscles. If you are on the lookout for a distinctive gift, you are in the right place. Let us continue this empowering journey together.

Methods for Focusing on Pelvic Muscles

Refining Your Focus

Once you've found your pelvic floor muscles, the next step is to focus on isolating and controlling them precisely. Being able to isolate these muscles is important for effective Kegel exercises and relieving symptoms of erectile dysfunction.

Mastering Isolation: The key is to contract and relax your pelvic floor muscles independently of nearby muscles. This precision is crucial for the success of Kegel exercises. Here are some ways to improve your focus:

Picture It: Close your eyes and picture your pelvic floor muscles. This is the place to get creative. Imagine the lifting and squeezing motion while concentrating solely on these muscles.

Breathe Right: Integrate controlled breathing into your routine. Inhale deeply, let your belly expand, and exhale with your pelvic floor muscles lifted and squeezed. Matching your breath to your exercise enhances muscle control and relaxation.

Go with the Flow: For better endurance, try rhythmic contractions. Gently contract your pelvic floor muscles, hold for a few seconds, and then gently relax. Repeat, gradually increasing the time for both contraction and relaxation.

Tech Assistance: Consider using biofeedback devices that give real-time feedback on your pelvic floor muscle activity. These gadgets offer visual or audio cues to help you understand how well your muscles are contracting and refine your technique.

Step by Step: Start with short, moderate contractions and progress to stronger, longer contractions as your muscle strength improves. This gradual approach promotes long-term development of pelvic floor strength.

Avoiding Common Mistakes:

Don't overdo it: Avoid excessive force during contractions to prevent muscle fatigue and potential injury.

Relaxation is key: Ensure full relaxation between contractions to avoid muscle tension and maintain flexibility.

Stay consistent: Establish a regular practice routine to strengthen muscle memory and maximize the benefits of isolation techniques.

Incorporating Techniques into Daily Life:

Integrate isolation strategies into your daily activities. Practice pelvic floor muscle contractions while working, driving, or watching TV to enhance muscle awareness and control over time.

Acknowledge Your Progress:

Perfecting pelvic floor muscle isolation takes time. Be patient and celebrate small victories, knowing that consistent effort will yield significant results.

You're laying the groundwork for a more focused and successful approach to Kegel exercises as you continue to enhance your ability to isolate and control your pelvic floor muscles. Section 4.3 will guide you through specific exercises to further improve muscle identification and isolation. Get ready to elevate your journey to address erectile dysfunction!

Exercises to Identify Muscles

Congrats on reaching this point! You've found and separated your pelvic floor muscles and learned to control them better. Now, let's do some exercises to identify muscles and get ready for more specialized Kegel exercises.

Exercise 1: Quick Contractions and Relaxations

Start with short squeezes and releases to improve your ability to quickly engage your pelvic floor muscles. Squeeze fast and relax for a few seconds. Repeat many times, increasing speed as you get more experience.

Exercise 2: Long Contractions

Try holding contractions for a longer time to build endurance and strengthen your pelvic floor muscles. Gradually increase the length of each squeeze, holding it as long as comfortable. This exercise is great for boosting muscle stamina over time.

Exercise 3: Breath-Coordinated Contractions

Time your contractions with your breath to enhance coordination and control. Inhale deeply, clench your pelvic floor muscles as you exhale, hold for a few seconds, and then inhale. This rhythmic syncing improves overall muscle awareness and strengthens the mind-body connection.

Exercise 4: Elevator Experiment

Imagine your pelvic floor muscles as an elevator going up and down. Tighten the muscles progressively with each floor, reaching max contraction on the top floor. Release gradually as the elevator falls. This exercise explores your pelvic floor muscles' full range of motion.

Exercise 5: Pelvic Floor Activation (Bridge Pose)

Add the bridge position to boost pelvic floor activation. Lie on your back, knees bent, and feet hip-width apart. Engage your pelvic floor muscles as you lift your hips. Hold for a few seconds before lowering your hips. This integrates muscle activation into a traditional workout, enhancing overall strength.

Exercise 6: Marching While Seated

Sit comfortably, feet flat on the ground. Lift one foot, activating your pelvic floor muscles. Return the foot and repeat on the other side. This seated marching exercise works pelvic floor muscles and improves stability and balance.

Exercise 7: Pelvic Tilts While Standing

Stand with feet shoulder-width apart. Gently tilt your pelvis forward and backward, focusing on pelvic floor muscle activation. This exercise enhances muscle control awareness in a weight-bearing position, simulating real-life conditions.

Progress at Your Own Pace

Remember, growth is personal. Start with easy exercises and gradually increase intensity and time as your strength develops. Consistency is key, so include these workouts in your daily routine.

You're actively improving your ability to recognize, isolate, and control your pelvic floor muscles with these exercises.

Chapter 5: Kegel Exercises: Beginner Level

These exercises, named after the esteemed Dr. Arnold Kegel, aim to fortify your pelvic floor muscles. Here, we will guide you through the rudiments of these exercises, ensuring not only comprehension but also fostering confidence in their regular integration into your routine.

Let's commence with the basics. The pelvic floor muscles constitute a network of tissues stretching from the pubic bone to the base of the spine, providing support to vital organs like the bladder and rectum. The weakening of these muscles can lead to issues such as erectile dysfunction. The silver lining is that with consistent engagement in these exercises, these muscles can be targeted and strengthened.

It's imperative to pinpoint the specific muscles involved. Initiate the process by identifying the muscles responsible for halting the flow of urine midstream. These are the muscles engaged during Kegel exercises. For optimal results and to minimize challenges, it's crucial to note that these exercises are best executed with an empty bladder.

Now, let's look into the exercises. Find a comfortable seated or reclined position. Inhale deeply, then contract your pelvic floor muscles for a count of three as you exhale. Visualize drawing these muscles upward and inward. Crucially, avoid engaging your abdomen, thighs, or buttocks during this sequence.

Sustain the contraction for a count of three, followed by a three-count release. Allow your muscles to return to their resting state completely between contractions. Initiate with ten repetitions, gradually escalating as familiarity with the routine grows.

Progression and customization are pivotal. Consistency is paramount as you embark on this journey. Start with a single set of ten repetitions daily and progressively increase to three sets. Should the identification of the appropriate muscles pose initial challenges, persevere; practice is key.

Now, let's touch upon the integration of these exercises into your routine. Consider incorporating them into your daily activities, perhaps aligning them with existing habits like tooth brushing. This way, they seamlessly become a natural part of your daily regimen, enhancing adherence.

For newcomers, initial muscular discomfort is anticipated and normal. It signifies the awakening and strengthening of your muscles. However, if discomfort persists, seeking medical attention is imperative.

Bear in mind that personal growth is a unique voyage. Celebrate even minor achievements, and resist the urge to hasten the process. Consistency and patience are your steadfast allies on the path to enhancing pelvic floor strength and overall sexual well-being.

Establishing a Routine

Now that you know the basics, let's talk about making a regular routine. The key to getting the most out of these exercises for your sexual health and overall well-being is to do them regularly.

The Importance of a Routine:

Think of your pelvic floor muscles like any other muscles in your body. They need regular, focused exercise to really get better. Having a routine not only helps you make Kegel exercises a habit, but it also ensures that you're taking care of your muscles.

Start by setting achievable goals. If you're just starting, commit to a certain number of sessions each week. It could be as simple as doing 10 minutes of Kegel exercises every day. As you get used to it, you can adjust the frequency and length to fit your schedule.

Incorporate into Daily Habits:

Try linking Kegel exercises to things you already do every day. Whether it's during your morning coffee, while watching TV, or before bed, connecting Kegels to a regular activity makes it easier to stick to your routine.

Using reminders can also help, especially in the beginning. Set alarms on your phone or put sticky notes in places where you'll see them to remind you to do your daily Kegel exercises. It's not just a little reminder; it also emphasizes how important it is to take care of your sexual health.

Track Your Progress:

Keeping track of your progress can motivate you along the way. Keep a simple diary to record your sessions each day or week. Note any improvements you notice, like increased stamina, better control, or positive changes in sexual function. This not only makes you feel successful but also helps you see patterns and areas where you can improve.

Overcoming Challenges:

Challenges are normal when you're trying to stay fit. Some days it might feel hard to stick to your routine because life gets busy, and there are many distractions. During those times, remind yourself of the long-term benefits. Think of Kegel exercises as an investment in your sexual health, and being consistent pays off in the end.

If you're struggling, consider finding a workout buddy for Kegel exercises. Sharing your journey with someone else adds a social aspect and gives you mutual support. You can share tips, celebrate achievements, and solve problems together.

Remember to be kind to yourself. If you miss a session or two, don't let guilt get in the way of your success. Recognize the setback and get back on track. This is about creating a lasting habit, and every effort counts.

Overcoming Challenges

Facing challenges is just a normal part of trying to do something awesome. Now, let's talk about common issues and how to solve them, so you can keep working towards fixing erectile dysfunction. Take it slow and steady:

Keeping up with your routine can be tough when life gets busy. Some days, finding time for Kegel exercises might feel hard. The key is to know that being consistent doesn't mean being perfect. If you miss a session, don't be too hard on yourself. Just get back to it and focus on sticking to your plan.

Handling Discomfort or Pain:

Starting Kegel exercises might make your muscles sore or uncomfortable. That's normal. But if the discomfort keeps going, you might need to change things up. Make sure you're working the right muscles and not accidentally using your belly or thighs. If the pain doesn't go away, talk to a healthcare provider or a pelvic floor physical therapist for personalized advice.

Staying Motivated:

Keeping motivated can be tough, especially after the initial excitement wears off. Set small goals and celebrate little achievements to keep going. Recognizing success, like doing more reps or having better muscle control, boosts your motivation. Remind yourself of the bigger benefits, like improved sexual function, bladder control, and overall pelvic health.

Dealing with Distractions:

Distractions are everywhere in our fast-paced world. Finding a quiet time for Kegel exercises can be tricky. Create a dedicated space for your routine to minimize interruptions. It could be a comfy spot at home or a peaceful place outside. Turning off electronic gadgets during exercises also helps you stay focused.

Spicing Up the Routine:

Repeating the same thing can get boring, and that's a motivation killer. To keep things interesting, try different Kegel exercises. Mix up your positions, try mindfulness techniques, or use guided pelvic floor workout apps. Adding variety prevents boredom and brings a fresh feel to your routine.

Getting Support:

Taking this journey alone can be scary. Consider getting help from your partner, friends, or joining online pelvic health communities. Sharing your experiences with others not only gives you support but also makes your journey feel more normal. Knowing that others are facing similar challenges can be really inspiring.

Adjusting the Routine:

Life changes, and so should your exercise plan. If your current schedule isn't working, be ready to make adjustments. Being flexible makes it easier to stick with it, whether you change the time of day or incorporate Kegels into other activities.

Remember, progress is the goal, not perfection. Every journey has challenges, and overcoming them adds up to your overall progress. When you tackle these obstacles, you're not just strengthening your pelvic muscles; you're also building resilience and dedication.

Chapter 6: Kegel Exercises: Intermediate Level

By now, you've probably mastered the basic exercises, building a strong foundation for your pelvic floor. In this chapter, we'll explore how to advance your Kegel practice for a smooth transition to more challenging techniques.

Building on Your Kegel Routine

It's important to remember the key principles as you move on to intermediate exercises. Kegels target the pelvic floor muscles, crucial for bladder control, sexual function, and overall pelvic support. The muscles you've been working on play a vital role in maintaining the bladder, rectum, and even erectile function.

Gradual Intensification: The intensity of intermediate Kegel exercises increases gradually. Instead of holding for the standard 5 seconds, try aiming for 7 to 10 seconds. This extended duration challenges your pelvic floor muscles, boosting strength and endurance.

Employing Resistance: Enhance the effectiveness of your Kegel workout by considering resistance. You can use specialized Kegel balls or pelvic floor weights for this purpose. These devices create resistance, making your muscles work harder. Start with lower resistance and progress as your strength builds.

Diversifying Your Routine: Add variety to your routine by doing Kegels in different positions. While sitting is a common choice, try standing or lying down as alternatives. Each position engages your muscles differently, providing a more comprehensive workout.

Professional Guidance: Consult a pelvic health physiotherapist or a healthcare professional experienced in pelvic floor rehabilitation. They can offer personalized advice based on your progress, ensuring you're on the right track and addressing any issues you may encounter.

Balancing Kegels and Relaxation: As you advance your Kegel routine, it's crucial to focus on relaxation. Taking breaks between contractions reduces muscle fatigue and enhances blood flow to the pelvic area. A well-rounded pelvic floor workout requires a careful balance of contraction and relaxation.

Tracking Your Progress: Keep a journal to document your workouts, noting the time, intensity, and any observations or sensations. This record is a valuable tool for both you and your healthcare provider, offering insights into your progress and helping tailor your routine for optimal results.

Patience and Consistency: Remember, improvement takes time. Be patient and stay committed to your efforts. Consistency is key to success with Kegel exercises. Celebrate both small and big achievements as you work towards better pelvic health and erectile function in the intermediate phase.

Advanced Methods To Enhance Pelvic Floor Strength

Here, we're going to explore more ways to strengthen your pelvic floor muscles and help with overcoming erectile dysfunction. Let's dive into these advanced techniques.

Extended Contractions: In this advanced stage, try holding your contractions for 10 to 15 seconds. This challenges your pelvic floor muscles to maintain tension for a longer time, making them stronger and more enduring, which is crucial for good pelvic health.

Pulse Contractions: Add quick, brief pulses after a prolonged contraction. This dynamic movement activates multiple muscle fibers in the pelvic floor, making your workout more challenging and helping your muscles adapt and grow stronger.

Eccentric Contractions: Instead of just focusing on the contraction, slowly release the tension after each one. This controlled release adds a new level of difficulty, promoting balanced strength and preventing muscular imbalances.

Dynamic Movements: Spice up your workout by combining Kegels with activities like squats or lunges. This simulates real-life scenarios where pelvic floor muscles are essential. Dynamic movements also improve coordination and stability.

Biofeedback Devices: Consider using these devices for real-time feedback on muscle activity. They help you target the right muscles and achieve optimal contractions, enhancing your technique and the effectiveness of your exercises.

Breathing Coordination: Sync your breathing with your Kegel exercises. Inhale deeply while relaxing your pelvic floor and exhale gently while contracting the muscles. This coordinated breathing enhances both muscle engagement and relaxation between contractions.

Resistance Training: Gradually increase resistance on your pelvic floor muscles as your strength improves. This can be done by raising the weight or resistance level of your tools. Progressive resistance keeps your muscles adapting and growing, preventing plateaus in your progress.

Personalized Approach: Customize your advanced Kegel program based on your specific needs. Pay attention to your body's responses and be willing to adjust your routine accordingly. This personalized approach ensures that you target specific areas while maximizing your efforts.

Remember, great rewards come from hard work. By embracing these advanced techniques, you're not just strengthening your pelvic floor but also making progress in overcoming erectile dysfunction.

Checking How You're Doing and What You've Achieved

As you work to improve erectile dysfunction, it's important to see and understand your progress. Let's explore some good ways to keep track of your progress and see the results of your focused Kegel program.

Regular Check-ins: Regularly checking in on yourself is an important part of tracking progress. Start by testing how strong and controlled your pelvic floor muscles are. Notice any changes or improvements in how strong and long your contractions are. Being aware of these changes is the foundation for effectively plotting your path.

Checking Erectile Function: One of the main goals of your Kegel exercises is to improve erectile function. Pay attention to any changes in how often and how well you get erections. You might see improvements in how stiff and lasting they are, indicating that your pelvic floor health is getting better. Feel free to tell your doctor about your observations if you want to know more.

Using Measures for Results: Include proven ways to measure results in your checking process. For example, the International Index of Erectile Function (IIEF) provides a structured way to assess erectile function. Doing these assessments regularly helps you track changes over time and gives useful information for discussions with healthcare experts.

Keeping Track of Pelvic Floor Symptoms: Note any pelvic floor symptoms you might have. Changes in how your bladder works, like better control, might mean your pelvic floor muscles are getting stronger. Also, less pelvic pain or discomfort shows good progress. Pay attention to these small changes because they affect your overall pelvic health.

Talking to Medical Professionals: Regular visits with healthcare experts are important for properly checking your progress. Share your findings, self-assessment results, and any concerns with your healthcare provider. They may give important insights, adjust your exercise routine as needed, and make sure you're on the right track to reaching your goals.

Changing Your Routine: Be ready to change your Kegel routine based on your progress and feedback from healthcare providers. This might mean adjusting how long or intense your exercises are, or trying new approaches. Being flexible ensures your routine adapts to your changing needs and goals.

Remembering Milestones: Celebrate both small and big achievements along the way. Recognizing improvements in endurance, better control, or positive changes in erectile function is important for staying motivated and dedicated to your Kegel exercises.

Keeping Records: Keep documenting your workouts, observations, and any changes to your program. Consistent documentation is a helpful tool during healthcare appointments, providing a full summary of your journey and allowing for informed discussions about your progress.

Chapter 7: Kegel Exercises: Advanced Level

In advanced Kegel exercises, we'll explore specific changes to help your pelvic floor health. Now that you've got the basics down, let's fine-tune your routine for even better results. These exercises focus on certain muscles in the pelvic floor, giving you a personalized approach to treating erectile dysfunction.

Let's begin with variations that target the pubococcygeus muscle (PC muscle), an important player in sexual function. Precise exercises can help strengthen the PC muscle, which plays a role in controlling urine flow and maintaining erectile function.

Isolated PC Muscle Contractions: Find a quiet spot to sit or lie comfortably. Take a few deep breaths to relax. Inhale and contract only your PC muscle, without involving other muscles. Exhale and release after a few seconds of holding the contraction. Repeat this for about ten times. This exercise isolates and targets the PC muscle, building strength and endurance. Over time, you'll gain better control over this crucial muscle, contributing to improved erectile function.

PC Muscle Staircase Contractions: Imagine your PC muscle as a multi-step ladder. Inhale and slightly contract the muscle, holding for a second. With each breath, increase the strength of the contraction, climbing the "staircase" of muscle activation. As you descend, gently release the tension after reaching the peak contraction. Repeat this pattern ten times. This method not only trains the PC muscle thoroughly but also enhances awareness and control. It's a gradual workout that stresses your pelvic floor.

Reverse Kegels for Balance: Traditional Kegel exercises involve clenching, while reverse Kegels focus on relaxation. Take a deep breath and sit comfortably. Exhale, intentionally relaxing your pelvic floor muscles as if letting go of stress. Practice this mild relaxation for ten breaths. Integrating reverse Kegels maintains balance in your pelvic floor, reducing excessive tightness. This can be especially effective for those unknowingly holding stress in their pelvic region, leading to erectile dysfunction.

Tailbone Tucks: Lie on your back with knees bent and feet flat. Inhale, then exhale, tilting your pelvis backward and tucking your tailbone toward the floor. Hold for a few seconds, feeling the pelvic floor engage. Inhale again, exhale, and let your tailbone return to neutral. Repeat ten times. Tailbone tucks add a dynamic aspect to your Kegel program, working various pelvic floor muscles and improving flexibility. This exercise promotes pelvic floor health by encouraging a larger range of motion.

Gradually add these variations to your Kegel routine, paying attention to your body's response. Remember, consistency is key. As you master these advanced exercises, you'll be on your way to a stronger, more resilient pelvic floor, addressing erectile dysfunction with precision and care.

Using Tools and Gadgets

Now, let's learn how equipment and gadgets can enhance your pelvic floor workout. You can make your workouts more effective by using special tools, adding a challenge and creativity to your routine. Let's check out some options:

Kegel Exercise Balls: These small, weighted spheres, also called Ben Wa balls, are designed to be inserted into the vagina. When you do Kegel exercises, the muscles naturally tighten around the balls, providing resistance and improving the workout. Start with lighter weights and progress to heavier ones as your pelvic floor strength improves. This increased resistance not only enhances muscle engagement but also improves your sense of your body's position.

Resistance Bands: Adding resistance bands to your Kegel exercises introduces external resistance, working your pelvic floor muscles in new ways. Loop one end of the band around your thighs and attach the other end to a secure point. The band adds resistance to Kegel contractions, requiring more effort from your pelvic floor muscles. It's especially effective for targeting the adductor muscles, contributing to a comprehensive pelvic floor workout.

Biofeedback Devices: Thanks to technology advancements, there are now biofeedback devices designed specifically for pelvic floor exercises. These gadgets provide real-time data on muscle activation, helping you engage the right muscles during exercises. Some devices use visual cues, while others use touch feedback. You can refine your technique with these tools, ensuring precise and efficient contractions. This increased awareness leads to improved pelvic floor function over time.

Smart Kegel Trainers: These interactive gadgets connect to smartphone apps to offer guided workouts and track progress. These trainers often include sensors that assess muscle strength and endurance. The app provides real-time feedback, making Kegel exercises more personalized and dynamic. Some apps even turn the workout into a game, adding a fun element to pelvic floor workouts.

Vibrating Pelvic Floor Massagers: These combine pleasure with function. The vibrations massage the pelvic floor muscles, promoting relaxation, and also trigger muscle contractions. This is particularly helpful for those who experience tightness or discomfort during Kegel exercises. Plus, the enjoyable sensations can help you develop a positive relationship with your pelvic floor training.

Take it slow and pay attention to how your body reacts when incorporating gadgets into your advanced Kegel routine. Ensure that any equipment you use is clean, safe, and suitable for your fitness level. By trying these new additions to your routine, you're not just exercising; you're embracing a personalized and dynamic approach to pelvic floor health that can assist with overcoming erectile dysfunction.

Tailoring Exercises to Fit Your Needs

When you start doing advanced Kegel exercises, you have lots of options to make them just right for you. This means you can adjust your pelvic floor workout to fit your own needs and challenges. As we go through this chapter, it's important to remember that everyone is different, and making these exercises work for you is the key to getting the most out of them. Let's explore how you can customize your advanced Kegel exercises for your specific needs:

Considering Age: As we get older, our muscles may change. If you're older, you can customize your Kegel exercises to match these changes. Focus on exercises that build endurance and hold your contractions for longer. Gradually increase how long you squeeze your muscles to test and strengthen your pelvic floor. Talk to a healthcare provider to make sure your routine is okay for any age-related health issues.

Customizing After Giving Birth: If you've recently had a baby, you might notice big changes in your pelvic floor. Start with simple exercises and gradually move on to more advanced ones to customize your postpartum Kegel exercises. Use diaphragmatic breathing to help your pelvic floor, and pay attention to any discomfort. Pelvic floor physical therapy can give you personalized advice and help you recover after giving birth.

Dealing with Health Issues and Surgeries: If you have certain health problems or have had pelvic surgery, you might need to adjust your Kegel exercises. It's important to talk to a healthcare provider, especially if you have issues like prostate problems or pelvic organ prolapse. They can help you modify your pelvic floor exercises to match your specific situation, making sure your routine supports your health.

Adding Other Exercises to Kegels: Think about combining Kegel exercises with other workouts to take care of your whole pelvic floor. Include exercises that strengthen your core, make your hips more flexible, and improve your overall heart health in your Kegel routine. Yoga and Pilates are good options because they work on your pelvic floor and boost your overall health.

Mind-Body Connection: Building a connection between your mind and body is an important part of customizing your Kegel exercises. Add mindfulness practices like meditation and visualization to your daily routine. When you do your exercises, focus on how your pelvic floor feels and imagine your muscles tightening and relaxing. This awareness not only makes your exercises more effective but also helps your overall well-being.

Staying Consistent and Monitoring Progress: You can customize your schedule and how you track your progress. Create a routine that fits into your daily life to make it easier to stick with. Keep track of your progress in a journal or with a fitness app, noting any improvements in muscle strength, endurance, or erectile function. Adjust your workouts as your needs change, and celebrate the small victories along the way.

Customizing advanced Kegel exercises to fit your needs is a freeing journey that recognizes how unique everyone's pelvic floor health is. By adjusting your routine based on your age, postpartum recovery, health issues, and overall well-being, you can not only address erectile dysfunction but also commit to a lifelong dedication to pelvic floor health and vitality.

"The power of Kegel exercises isn't defined by noise or fanfare but by the quiet commitment that fosters a renewed sense of confidence and inner strength."

Chapter 8: Lifestyle Factors and ED

The way someone lives can greatly affect the chances of them having trouble in the bedroom. Things like what they eat, how active they are, how stressed they feel, and the drugs they use can directly affect the health of their blood vessels and hormones. These are really important for being able to perform sexually. Knowing how lifestyle choices connect to these issues helps us see how our everyday actions can impact our sexual health.

How Your Diet Affects Your Ability to Have a Good Time in the Bedroom

Just like your heart needs good food to function at its best, another important part of your body—responsible for close encounters—does too.

Let's dive into the details. Eating nutritious food is not only good for your overall health but can also have a big impact on your sex life. Antioxidants play a major role in this nutritional performance. These powerful ingredients fight stress in your body that can affect blood flow, which is crucial for intimate performance.

Think of your blood arteries as roads that carry supplies to different parts of your body, especially the one that matters most in intimate moments. Antioxidants, found in colorful fruits and veggies like berries, spinach, and tomatoes, act like traffic police, ensuring smooth blood flow.

Omega-3 fatty acids are another hero in this story. These healthy fats, found in fish like salmon and trout, as well as in flaxseeds and walnuts, support good blood circulation and keep your arteries flexible. Think of them as the oil for your internal roads, preventing any blockages.

And don't forget the importance of staying hydrated. Water is essential for life, and being well-hydrated is crucial for overall health, including sexual function. Proper hydration keeps your blood volume up and helps prevent issues related to dehydration that might affect your ability to perform.

Now, let's talk about the not-so-friendly fats, saturated and trans fats. These are like the bad guys on the roads, blocking your arteries and stopping blood flow. Cutting down on saturated fats found in fried foods and processed snacks, as well as avoiding trans fats often found in baked goods, is a key step to improve vascular health and, consequently, intimate performance.

Your diet is crucial for a strong foundation in intimate health. Think of it as fueling your body's engine for optimal performance. Include a variety of fruits and veggies, omega-3-rich foods, and stay hydrated. These dietary changes not only boost your overall health but also contribute to enjoyable and satisfying personal moments.

Exercise, Weight, and Erectile Health

Let's put on our imaginary sneakers and step into the topic of exercise, managing weight, and how they impact erectile health. Now that we've learned how food affects our intimate well-being, let's chat about moving our bodies.

Think of exercise as the heartbeat of a healthy life—it pumps energy all over, even to your private parts. Doing regular exercise has some perks for your ability to get and keep an erection. It helps blood flow, which is super important for an erection.

Activities like brisk walking, jogging, or biking get your blood flowing, even down there. This is good for both your ability to get hard and your overall heart health—a win-win!

Now, let's talk about lifting weights. It helps tone your muscles, especially the ones you use during sexy time. Tonier muscles mean you can have and keep erections better, just like a strong core helps.

Moving on to exercise and weight control. Keeping a healthy weight is crucial for good erectile health. Carrying extra weight, especially around your belly, can cause problems like insulin resistance and inflammation. These can mess with blood vessels and testosterone levels, both key players in a good time in bed.

Exercise isn't just for losing weight; it helps you keep it off too. You don't need intense workouts. Find things you like and make them a regular part of your day. It's about making exercise enjoyable and doable every day.

Now, let's tackle the big issue: erectile dysfunction and how it connects to your mind. Exercise is like a natural stress-reliever and mood booster. It makes your body produce endorphins, which are feel-good chemicals that help with stress and anxiety. Taking care of your physical and mental health is key because stress and bad mental health can really mess with your ability to get it up.

Lastly, think of exercise as a way to celebrate what your body can do. Find activities you enjoy, whether it's dancing, swimming, or hitting the gym, and make them a regular thing. Remember, every step, lift, and minute of exercise is an investment in your sexual health and overall well-being. So, lace up those shoes, enjoy moving around, and see your intimate health thrive!

Stress, Sleep, and their Impact on ED

Now that we've taken care of our bodies with a balanced diet and exercise, let's explore how stress and sleep can significantly affect erectile performance. These often overlooked aspects of our lives play a crucial role in the intricate dynamics of intimacy.

To begin, stress is a constant companion in our fast-paced lives. It's not just a mental burden; it also has physical effects on various body systems, including those related to sexual wellness. Chronic stress can lead to elevated levels of cortisol, the primary stress hormone in the body. This hormonal imbalance can disrupt the precise interplay of neurotransmitters and blood flow necessary for a healthy erection.

Think of stress as a detour on the path to intimacy. It causes congestion, hindering the smooth flow of messages and blood to the crucial areas. Managing stress isn't a luxury; it's a necessity for maintaining good sexual health. Incorporate stress-relieving activities into your daily routine, such as mindfulness meditation, deep breathing exercises, or engaging in joyful hobbies. By doing so, you're not only enhancing your mental well-being but also creating a conducive environment for enjoyable personal moments.

Now, let's shift our focus to sleep—a critical component of overall health and well-being. During sleep, your body undergoes healing processes, including those related to sexual function. Insufficient sleep can lead to decreased testosterone levels, hormonal imbalances, and feelings of tiredness and irritation, all detrimental to meaningful connections.

Consider sleep as your body's reset button. During these peaceful hours, your system recharges, preparing you physically and mentally for the challenges of the day ahead.

Aim for 7-9 hours of quality sleep each night to provide your body with ample time for the intricate dance of repair and regeneration.

It's crucial to establish a sleep-friendly environment. Maintain a dark, quiet, and cool bedroom, and disconnect from electronic devices at least an hour before bedtime to signal to your body that it's time to unwind.

Sometimes, it's tough dealing with the issues that comes with Erectile Dysfunction, but you have the assurance that it can be defeated. Others have conquered it, and so will you.

Chapter 9: Complementary Therapies

Complementary therapies are different kinds of treatments that are not typically used by doctors. They aim to make people feel better in addition to regular medical treatments. For Erectile Dysfunction (ED), these treatments often look into different methods like acupuncture, herbal supplements, and lifestyle changes. The goal is to improve the regular treatments or deal with the reasons behind ED. These alternative methods may give extra help and possible benefits for people dealing with ED, even though how well they work can be different for each person.

Acupuncture and Erectile Dysfunction

Acupuncture is an ancient Chinese medicine technique that's become popular for helping with various health issues, including erectile dysfunction (ED). In this method, tiny needles are inserted into specific places on the body to improve energy flow and overall well-being.

People think acupuncture helps with ED by boosting blood circulation, reducing stress, and balancing the body's energy channels. According to Chinese medicine, issues with the flow of Qi, the body's essential energy, can lead to sexual health problems, and acupuncture aims to fix these imbalances.

Understanding how acupuncture works is important before thinking about it as a therapy for ED. During a session, a licensed practitioner delicately inserts needles into specific acupoints on the body. These acupoints are said to be connected to energy pathways called meridians. Stimulating these areas is believed to restore balance and improve the overall function of various organs, including those involved in sexual wellness.

Studies have looked into the potential benefits of acupuncture for ED. One study in the International Journal of Impotence Research found that men who received acupuncture had better erectile function than those who didn't. This improvement may be due to increased blood flow to the genital region and lower stress levels.

In Western medicine, acupuncture may affect the release of neurotransmitters and hormones like endorphins and serotonin, which impact mood and stress. By influencing these elements, acupuncture may lead to a more relaxed state and improved sexual function.

It's important to note that when done by a skilled and experienced practitioner, acupuncture is generally considered safe.

Individual reactions may vary, so it's wise to talk to a healthcare practitioner before considering acupuncture as a supplementary therapy for ED.

Apart from acupuncture, lifestyle factors play a crucial role in treating ED. A comprehensive approach to sexual health involves regular exercise, a balanced diet, and stress management. When combined with these lifestyle changes, acupuncture may offer a holistic approach to maintaining erectile function.

As a supplementary therapy for ED, acupuncture may help restore erectile function by improving blood circulation, reducing stress, and balancing the body's energy channels. While research on acupuncture and ED continues, positive results have been found, and many people consider it a beneficial addition to their overall approach to sexual health.

Yoga and Meditation for Erectile Health

Yoga and meditation have become powerful tools for achieving overall well-being and enhancing sexual health. These practices go beyond the common associations with flexibility and stress relief, offering a holistic approach to addressing both the physical and psychological aspects of erectile dysfunction (ED).

Yoga

Originating from ancient Indian philosophy, yoga combines physical postures, controlled breathing, and meditation. Certain yoga positions, such as Downward-Facing Dog, Cobra, and Bridge Pose, play a crucial role in improving blood circulation, flexibility, and strength—key components of sexual well-being. These poses specifically target pelvic muscles, enhancing blood flow to the genital region.

Yoga not only benefits the body but also contributes to mental and emotional well-being. By providing a disciplined method for reducing stress, anxiety, and depression—the major contributors to ED—yoga fosters a mind-body connection. Mindfulness, a central aspect of yoga, increases awareness of this link, promoting relaxation and minimizing the impact of stress on sexual function.

Meditation

Frequently paired with yoga, meditation offers another effective strategy for improving erectile health. Mindfulness meditation involves concentrating on the present moment without judgment, aiding in managing stress, worry, and negative thought patterns associated with sexual dysfunction.

Research indicates that daily meditation can positively affect various physiological markers linked to ED. It may help reduce cortisol, a stress hormone that can interfere with testosterone synthesis and contribute to sexual issues. Additionally, meditation has been associated with enhanced nitric oxide synthesis, a chemical that relaxes blood vessels and promotes blood flow—an essential factor in establishing and maintaining an erection.

Integrating Yoga and Meditation into Daily Life

Incorporating yoga and meditation into one's lifestyle doesn't require a significant time commitment. Short, targeted sessions tailored to individual preferences and schedules can have a substantial impact. Consistency is key, whether performing a few yoga postures before bedtime or engaging in a brief meditation session during the day.

The accessibility of online materials and seminars makes it easier than ever to explore and adopt these practices. Guided programs catering to beginners introduce them to yoga postures and meditation methods in a gentle manner. Thanks to this accessibility, individuals can embark on their journey toward improved erectile health at their own pace.

By incorporating specific yoga poses and mindfulness meditation into one's routine, individuals can enhance blood circulation, flexibility, and mental well-being. These practices aid in managing stress, worry, and negative thought patterns that may contribute to sexual problems. As with any complementary treatment, it's advisable to consult with a healthcare practitioner before introducing yoga and meditation into your routine to ensure a safe and personalized approach to improving erectile health.

Exploring Supplements for Erectile Dysfunction

Our focus turns to supplements—comprising vitamins, minerals, herbs, and natural components. In a market saturated with products claiming to enhance sexual health, understanding the science behind supplements and their potential role in treating ED is crucial for making well-informed decisions.

L-Arginine and Nitric Oxide Production

Let's start with L-Arginine, an amino acid found in certain foods and available as a supplement. It plays a vital role in the generation of nitric oxide, a vasodilator that relaxes blood vessels, facilitating increased blood flow. In the context of ED, sufficient blood flow to the penis is essential for achieving and sustaining an erection.

Research suggests that L-Arginine supplementation may boost nitric oxide synthesis, thereby enhancing blood circulation and potentially alleviating symptoms of mild to moderate ED. However, individual reactions to L-Arginine can vary, emphasizing the importance of consulting with a healthcare expert, particularly for individuals with pre-existing medical conditions.

Ginseng

Now, let's explore ginseng, an adaptogenic herb derived from various plant roots with a rich history in traditional medicine. This plant is believed to aid the body in adapting to stress and promoting overall vitality, including sexual health. Numerous studies have investigated the potential benefits of ginseng in improving erectile function.

According to a study in the International Journal of Impotence Research, ginseng may increase nitric oxide production and enhance overall sexual satisfaction. While these findings are promising, caution is advised, as further research is needed to establish the effectiveness and safety of ginseng as an ED therapy.

Zinc

Zinc is an essential mineral crucial for various bodily functions, including reproductive health. Zinc is involved in the production of testosterone, a hormone essential for male sexual activity. Some studies indicate a connection between zinc deficiency and sexual dysfunction.

Zinc supplementation may be beneficial for those deficient in this mineral, but it's crucial to strike a balance, as excessive zinc intake can be harmful. Consulting with a healthcare expert is advisable to determine individual needs and appropriate doses.

Tribulus Terrestris

Our exploration of complementary therapies concludes with tribulus terrestris, a plant traditionally used in herbal medicine, garnering attention for its potential role in improving sexual function. Some research suggests that this plant may elevate testosterone levels and contribute to sexual well-being.

Exercising caution is crucial when considering tribulus terrestris due to limited research and variations in product quality; therefore, consulting with a healthcare expert before incorporating it into your routine is advised for safe and effective usage, considering individual reactions and tailoring the approach to your unique needs and health status.

Chapter 10: Maintaining Erectile Health

Keeping your erectile health in good shape involves a mix of lifestyle choices and careful healthcare steps. Eating well, staying active, and managing stress all play a role in keeping your blood flow and nerves working well for the long run. It's also important to quickly address any other health issues you might have and ditch habits like smoking and drinking too much, as they can seriously affect your long-term erectile health.

Taking the Long-Term Path with Kegel Exercises

These exercises are crucial for keeping your ability to have erections healthy. We've talked about the good things Kegels can do in this book. They not only help with fixing issues but also stop them from happening. Now, we'll talk about why it's important to make Kegels a regular part of your routine for keeping your sexual health good over a long time.

Understanding the Long-Term Benefit

Doing Kegel exercises isn't a quick fix; it's something you need to keep doing for a long time. If you do them regularly, they help make the muscles in your pelvic floor healthy. These muscles support the bladder, rectum, and play a part in having erections. Regular exercise helps these muscles get stronger and last longer, improving blood flow and nerves in the pelvic area.

Preventing Erectile Issues: One big advantage of doing Kegel exercises for a long time is avoiding problems with erections. By keeping your pelvic floor muscles healthy, you're building a strong foundation for good long-term performance. These exercises act like a shield, stopping potential problems before they get serious and making sure blood flows well to the tissues that help with erections.

Adding Variety to Your Routine: To keep doing Kegel exercises for a long time, it helps to make them interesting and different. Just like any workout plan, doing the same thing every time can get boring. Try changing how long you do the exercises, how hard you do them, or even try different types of contractions. This not only challenges your muscles but also keeps you excited to keep up with your routine.

Staying Regular: Doing Kegel exercises regularly is super important for any long-term health plan. Make it a must-do in your daily routine. Find a time that works for you, whether it's in the morning, during lunch, or before bed, and stick to it. Being consistent helps your muscles remember what to do and makes sure doing Kegels becomes a normal part of your life.

The Emotional Side: Doing Kegel exercises for a long time is not just about keeping your body healthy; it's also about feeling good mentally. Doing exercises that help with erections should be part of your routine to boost your confidence and feel good about yourself. People often forget about this emotional side, but it's a big part of staying sexually healthy.

In the end, committing to doing Kegel exercises for a long time is like investing in your sexual health and overall well-being. If you keep doing them regularly, mix things up, and pay attention, you not only avoid issues with erections but also make your personal life better and more satisfying. So, let's continue this journey together to make sure your pelvic floor muscles stay strong and healthy for many years.

Making Kegels a Habit in Daily Life

Turning Kegels into a habit doesn't need to be a big challenge; it can actually be a pretty fun and easy thing that's good for your health overall.

Getting Kegels into Your Daily Routine: Kegel exercises are like chameleons—they can fit into different situations. You don't need a special spot or fancy gear. Try doing Kegels while you're at work, on your way to places, or even while watching TV. Since these exercises are quiet, you can do them without anyone noticing, making them a breeze to squeeze into your busy day.

Mindful Moments: Doing Kegels isn't just about going through the motions; it's also about tuning in to your body. Pay attention to how your muscles feel when you're doing Kegels. Being aware not only makes your exercises work better but also helps your brain connect the action with the good stuff it does for your sexual health.

Set Those Reminders: With life buzzing around, it's easy to forget about your health. Use your phone to remind yourself to do Kegels. Connect it to something you already do, like brushing your teeth or having your morning coffee. Regular reminders help turn Kegels into a habit, making it more likely you'll stick with it.

Mixing Kegels with Other Exercises: If you're already into fitness, try adding Kegels to your routine. They can team up with other exercises to boost your pelvic floor strength. Sneak in pelvic floor squeezes during aerobics, lifting weights, or yoga for a well-rounded approach to your health.

Team Up: Turn Kegels into a teamwork thing with your partner. Sync up your Kegel routines to make sexual health a shared goal. It not only deepens your connection but also gives you both a buddy system to stick to your routines.

Celebrating to Achievements: Celebrate the wins along the way as you bring Kegels into your daily life. Whether it's hitting a time goal or feeling those muscles getting stronger, acknowledging your success makes the positive impact even better. Celebrating victories also gives you a boost to keep up with your Kegel game.

Getting Help from the Pros

Talking to professionals is a smart step in keeping your sexual health in check with Kegel exercises. While doing Kegels on your own is usually fine, having a chat with a healthcare expert or a specialist can give you helpful tips, sort out any issues, and make sure you're doing things right for the best results.

Why Professional Advice Matters: When it comes to exercises for your pelvic floor, knowing your health details is crucial. Getting help from a pro lets you have a plan that fits your specific situation, considering any health issues, past surgeries, or other things that might affect your pelvic floor. A healthcare expert, like a urologist, physiotherapist, or sexual health pro, can help you shape up your Kegel routine.

Assessment and Plans Just for You: Pros can check how your pelvic floor muscles are doing right now. They might do tests or exams to find out if there are any weak spots or imbalances. Based on what they find, they can make a Kegel exercise plan that hones in on specific areas that need attention while avoiding possible problems.

Doing It Right: Even though Kegels seem simple, doing them the right way is super important. Pros can make sure you're doing the exercises correctly, so you get the most benefits without risking harm. Messing up Kegels could lead to not-so-great results or make existing problems worse, so it's wise to seek professional help.

Dealing with Erectile Issues: If you're dealing with erectile dysfunction, talking to a pro becomes even more crucial. A healthcare expert can help figure out what's causing the problem and suggest a full plan that might include Kegels and other treatments. Whether it's related to blood flow, nerves, or mental stuff, they've got you covered.

Keeping Tabs on Progress: Regular check-ins with a healthcare expert let them keep an eye on how you're doing. They can track your progress, tweak your Kegel routine if needed, and deal with any new issues as soon as they pop up. This team effort makes sure you're not facing sexual health challenges alone but with the support and know-how of a skilled pro.

Mixing It Up: Sometimes, Kegels are just one piece of the puzzle. Pros might suggest other things like lifestyle changes or dietary tweaks to boost your overall sexual health. Combining different treatments under professional guidance gives a well-rounded approach to tackling sexual health issues.

Emotional Support and Learning: Seeking help from pros doesn't just cover the physical stuff—it's there for your emotions too. Dealing with sexual health problems can be tough, but specialists can offer support, comfort, and tools to help you feel better overall. Learning about how mental health and erectile function are connected is also part of the package when you get professional help.

Conclusion

Thanks for joining in on our exploration of Kegel exercises and how they can do wonders for treating erectile dysfunction. Your commitment to understanding and using this important information is commendable. Keep in mind that just knowing the facts won't change you; it's the consistent practice that makes a difference.

As you wrap up this read, I encourage you to embark on the path to pelvic health with enthusiasm. To get the best results, perform these exercises diligently and make them a part of your routine. Your persistence will lay the foundation for stronger pelvic muscles and possibly improved erectile function.

If this journey has sparked your interest, consider checking out some of my other works. There's a wealth of content out there, each piece aiming to offer insights and ideas for living a fitter, better, and happier life.

Thanks once again for sharing your time and attention with me. May your quest for better pelvic health and overall well-being be marked by continuous growth and success.

BONUS

Instructions

Date: Fill in the date of your workout.

Exercise Routine: Write down the specific Kegel exercises you did in the session.

Duration: Note how much time each exercise or the entire session took.

Observations/Challenges: While working out, jot down any observations, problems, improvements, or other important notes.

Make it a habit to use this journal regularly for keeping tabs on your Kegel exercises. Record the activities, their durations, and any observations or obstacles during each session. This journal will help you monitor consistency, progress, and any adjustments needed in your routine.

DATE	EXERCISE ROUTINE	DURATION	OBSERVATION

DATE	EXERCISE ROUTINE	DURATION	OBSERVATION

DATE	EXERCISE ROUTINE	DURATION	OBSERVATION

DATE	EXERCISE ROUTINE	DURATION	OBSERVATION

DATE	EXERCISE ROUTINE	DURATION	OBSERVATION

DATE	EXERCISE ROUTINE	DURATION	OBSERVATION

DATE	EXERCISE ROUTINE	DURATION	OBSERVATION

DATE	EXERCISE ROUTINE	DURATION	OBSERVATION

DATE	EXERCISE ROUTINE	DURATION	OBSERVATION

www.ingramcontent.com/pod-product-compliance
Lightning Source LLC
Chambersburg PA
CBHW070806260726
48660CB00005B/1726